A 42-Day Devotional
in Company *with*
Henri J. M. Nouwen

Hope

for

Caregivers

Edited by Susan Martins Miller

ĩvp

An imprint of InterVarsity Press
Downers Grove, Illinois

InterVarsity Press
P.O. Box 1400 | Downers Grove, IL 60515-1426
ivpress.com | email@ivpress.com

InterVarsity Press® is the publishing division of InterVarsity Christian Fellowship/USA®.
For more information, visit intervarsity.org.

Scripture quotations, unless otherwise noted, are from the New Revised Standard Version Bible, copyright © 1989 National Council of the Churches of Christ in the United States of America. Used by permission. All rights reserved worldwide.

While any stories in this book are true, some names and identifying information may have been changed to protect the privacy of individuals.

The publisher cannot verify the accuracy or functionality of website URLs used in this book beyond the date of publication.

Cover design and image composite: David Fassett

ISBN 978-1-5140-0554-5 (hardcover) | ISBN 978-1-5140-1587-2 (paperback) |
ISBN 978-1-5140-0555-2 (digital)

Printed in the United States of America ♾

Library of Congress Cataloging-in-Publication Data
Names: Nouwen, Henri J. M., author.
Title: Hope for caregivers : a 42-day devotional in company with Henri J. M. Nouwen / Henri J. M. Nouwen.
Description: Downers Grove. Illinois : IVP, an imprint of InterVarsity Press, 2022. | Includes
  bibliographical references.
Identifiers: LCCN 2022013784 (print) | LCCN 2022013785 (ebook) | ISBN 9781514005545 (hardcover)
  | ISBN 9781514005552 (ebook)
Subjects: LCSH: Caregivers–Religious life. | Devotional literature.
Classification: LCC BV4910.9 .N678 2022 (print) | LCC BV4910.9 (ebook) | DDC 242/.4–dc23/
  eng/20220603
LC record available at https://lccn.loc.gov/2022013784
LC ebook record available at https://lccn.loc.gov/2022013785

34 33 32 31 30 29 28 27 26 | 13 12 11 10 9 8 7 6 5 4 3

"Henri Nouwen's words of consolation and wisdom are found in this precious book for caregivers—which includes each of us in relationship with others who suffer from debilitating illnesses. We often experience caregiving as tiring and burdensome, but Henri offers another vision that is lived more from the heart. Here he offers caregivers inspirational words about care—one for each day—for forty-two days. Resolving to remember only one point about 'heart-caring' throughout our workday will not only enhance the lives of those we care for but will also inspire our desire for healing in those who suffer."

Sue Mosteller, CSJ, executor of Henri Nouwen's literary estate

"This gentle book has a place close by my spot for renewal and rest. Each daily reflection never fails to take me to a quiet place of meditation, insight, and strength for the day. Each reading contains guidance from Holy Scripture, an insight from Henri, and a few thoughts to help you renew your perspective for love and care."

Lorna Dueck, consultant and caregiver for the Parkinson's disease journey

"Caregiving can be a difficult role, whether you are a family caregiver or care for others in the workplace. *Hope for Caregivers* is a wonderful compilation of sacred Scripture and the wisdom of beloved spiritual writer Henri Nouwen. This beautiful book is sure to support and inspire caregivers in any setting. Published as a six-week devotional and filled with questions to ponder, it can easily be used for personal reflection or in a group setting."

Michelle O'Rourke, author of *Healthy Caregiving: Perspectives for Caring Professionals in Company with Henri J. M. Nouwen*

"Caregiving is the holy act of the literal laying of hands on another to help and to heal. It requires strength, courage, and commitment to serve another intimately with dignity, respect, and love. The giving of such care, however, gives the one who cares a glimpse into God's priceless kenotic gift to humanity. This beautiful and important devotional based on Nouwen's magnanimous wisdom offers encouragement to those entrusted with caregiving by reminding them that what they are doing plants roots in the eternal—even in the hidden or lonely recesses of servitude, caregivers are seen, they matter, and they are upheld by the right hand of God!"

Carolyn Weber, caregiver, professor of literature, and author of *Surprised by Oxford*

"Caregivers are steady sources of grace, mercy, and truth—but who cares for the caregivers? Who affirms the work that they do and cheers them on? The devotionals in this book taken from the writings of Henri Nouwen offer guidance and inspiration, each day's reading bringing life-giving insight for the caregiver."

Mel Lawrenz, author of *A Chronicle of Grief: Finding Life After Traumatic Loss*

Contents

Introduction

MORE THAN 20 YEARS AFTER HIS DEATH, Henri Nouwen's life and writings on the spiritual life continue to touch millions of people in dozens of languages. Henri was born in the Netherlands in 1932 and was drawn to the priesthood in the Catholic church at a young age. After being ordained in 1957, he undertook further studies in psychology in the United States. In 1966 he accepted a position teaching psychology at the University of Notre Dame and wrote his first two books while there.

After earning a doctorate in theology, Henri spent ten years on the faculty of Yale Divinity School, where his classes were some of the most popular on campus. During these years, he also was publishing prolifically. Later, Henri became interested in Latin America and the many poor affected by both political turmoil and theological developments. For a time, he considered living and ministering in Peru.

Instead of Latin America, Henri accepted a position on the faculty at Harvard, but he remained restless. Despite the outward trappings of success

> *He had a way of making every person feel as if he or she were the only thing that mattered, regardless of what else was going on.*

as a professor and author, Henri struggled with depression and yearned for deeper meaning and personal connection with others. A chance meeting with Jean Vanier, the founder of L'Arche, an international movement of communities that welcome people living with disabilities, changed the path of Henri's life, and he moved to Daybreak, a L'Arche community near Toronto in Canada. He served in a pastoral role, gave countless talks and retreats, welcomed hundreds who sought counsel, and still found time to write, eventually publishing over 40 books. He lived in a community setting, where those living with disabilities and those caring for them shared life together. Henri was asked to care for Adam, a man with severe disability. At Daybreak he felt he had at last come home, and he spent the final ten years of his life there.

Henri suffered a heart attack in 1996 and was buried close to his beloved Daybreak community. His legacy lived on in the work of the Henri Nouwen Society, the Henri Nouwen Trust, and the Henri J. M. Nouwen Archives and Research Collection and in the enduring values of compassion, community and ministry that shine through all his writings.

A LIVING LEGACY

During the ten years Henri spent at Yale, Dr. Scott Morris was a student in the divinity school, enrolled in courses Henri taught, served on a faculty-student committee with him, and attended compline services Henri led each day. As he wrestled with his own calling to establish a church-based health center at some point in the future, Dr. Morris even went for a week of silence in the Taize community in France at Henri's suggestion. After he graduated from Yale and went on to medical school, Dr. Morris only ever saw Henri one other time. He'd heard Henri would be speaking near where he lived and made the effort to attend the event and to speak to Henri afterward. As was characteristic for Henri, he opened his arms wide for his former student. He had a way of making every person feel as if he or she were the only thing that mattered, regardless of what else was going on.

Dr. Morris completed both his theological and medical studies, moved to Memphis because it was one of the poorest cities in the country, and opened a faith-based organization to provide health care to people working in low-wage jobs without insurance or with inadequate insurance.

In 2016, a rare opportunity brought Henri Nouwen and Scott Morris back together again, when Karen Pascal, executive director of the Henri Nouwen Society and Legacy Trust, became interested in the work of

Caregiving is full of stories, and sometimes we need somebody to walk with us— someone who knows us well and whom we trust with parts of our stories that most people will never hear.

Church Health, which is still caring for people in low-wage jobs 30 years later. In addition, Church Health publishes resources around themes of faith and health. Conversations turned to the topic of caregiving, which both brought Henri his deepest spiritual joy and is an ever-growing need among individuals and faith communities that Church Health reaches across the nation.

Church Health and Henri Nouwen Society and Legacy Trust have partnered to create resources that address the needs of people in caregiving roles, whether that be caring for a child with special needs, a family member with chronic illness, an aging parent, someone struggling for mental health, or any other role that requires an individual to step out of awareness primarily of the individual's needs and into the circle of understanding of the care receiver's needs. This was a topic close to Henri's heart and shows up in many of his writings.

It is our deep joy to offer *Hope for Caregivers*, six weeks of daily devotionals that feature themes in Henri Nouwen's personal letters and published writings paired with Scripture passages and brief reflections and prayers for caregivers.

CARING WITH HOPE

These daily devotionals are arranged around six themes:

1. The eyes of pain—we see you.

2. Our greatest gift—you are doing something hard.

3. An invitation to joy—the experience will change you.

4. The prayer of caring—you are not alone.

5. The voice of love—you are God's beloved.

6. Rise to new life—love triumphs.

Each week, a letter that Henri wrote in his personal correspondence shows his understanding of the taxing issues of being a caregiver and sets the tone for the meditations that follow. Start each day's reading with a nugget of insight from Henri Nouwen. A Scripture verse follows, as well as a few lines of reflection and questions that weave together Henri's insight and the verse to offer encouragement and self-understanding even if all you have is a few minutes to ponder these thoughts. Wrap up with a sentence prayer. Maybe there are days when you can't find the words to pray, but the prayer of the devotional can be your own.

Hope for Caregivers works well for private reading and reflection. Caregiving is full of stories, and sometimes we need somebody to walk with us—someone who knows us well and whom we trust with parts of our stories that most people will never hear. If you have a companion like that in your life, *Hope for Caregivers* might be something that you'd like to read together. Even if geography or responsibilities do not allow you to be physically together every day, you can read separately and then share reflections and encouragement on the phone or in an e-mail by using the reflection questions to spur your thoughts and the prayer as a reminder to pray for each other.

Another way to use *Hope for Caregivers* is in a support group setting. We realize it's unlikely that a group of caregivers can meet in person every day for six weeks. However, it might be an encouragement to the whole group to know that others are reading the same devotions and wrestling with the same questions. Then when you are face-to-face, you have a basis for your sharing and discussion. Even if not everyone is reading along at the same pace, if you lead a support group, you might like to flag devotions that you feel are especially pertinent to the people in your group.

No matter how you choose to use *Hope for Caregivers*—individually, with a friend, or in a group—our prayer is that it brings you encouragement in finding meaning and significance in your caregiving relationships.

You are God's beloved. Never forget.

*Start your
story here*

WEEK 1

The Eyes of Pain

Much of caregiving is unseen by anyone but the caregiver, who may also feel unseen. The experience of caregiving becomes a lens for seeing life.

THIS WEEK CONSIDER THIS QUESTION

What is your story of seeing and being seen as a caregiver?

AFTER READING YOUR VERY pain-filled but also very grace-filled letter, I had only one desire—to come visit you. More than anything I wanted to spend some time with you, to offer you my love and friendship and to learn from you who has been tempted so much. I realize that I cannot come to you and you cannot come to me.

I simply want to ask you to trust that the Lord will continue to give you the strength to live through your pains with your husband and your son. Your letter shows that you have a great faith, courage and confidence, even though you yourself do not feel it as much. But God has not left you alone. I am sure that he will give you all the strength you need to be faithful in the midst of your agony.

love
Henri

THE HEART OF BEING HUMAN

In the realm of the Spirit of God, living and caring are one. Our society suggests that caring and living are quite separate and that caring belongs primarily to professionals who have received special training. Although training is important, and although certain people need preparation to practice their profession with competence, caring is a privilege of every person and is at the heart of being human. When we look at the original meaning of the word profession and realize the term refers, first of all, to professing one's own deepest conviction, then the essential spiritual unity between living and caring becomes clear. I look at care as helping others to claim for themselves the spiritual truth that they are—as we are—children of God, brothers and sisters of each other, and parents of generations to come.

Henri J. M. Nouwen

God's love was revealed among us in this way: God sent his only Son into the world so that we might live through him. In this is love, not that we loved God but that he loved us and sent his Son to be the atoning sacrifice for our sins. Beloved, since God loved us so much, we also ought to love one another.

—1 JOHN 4:9–11

REFLECTION

Offering care easily becomes reduced to tasks—the sometimes unpleasant activities that the care receiver cannot do independently. But that is a detached mindset. Caregiving as a calling or privilege is not rooted in tasks but in connection between human beings. The writer of 1 John tells us that this connection is through love, first from God and then through us as we see each other as human beings all beloved by God. Through love, living and caring are one.

- How do you respond to the idea of caregiving as a privilege at the heart of being human?
- What has been your most privileged moment in your caregiving story?

God of generations to come, show the realm of your Spirit and fill your people with overflowing love in the unseen moments of caring. Amen.

LISTENING FOR GOD

The word obedience *includes the Latin word* audire, *which means "listening."*
Living a spiritually mature life is living a life in which we listen to the voice of
God's Spirit within and among us and in which we try to respond to that voice at
every moment of our lives. The great news of God's revelation is not simply that
God exists, but also that God is actively present in our lives at all times and in all
places. Our God is a God who cares, heals, guides, directs, challenges, confronts,
and corrects us. He is a God who wants to lead us closer to the full realization
of our humanity. To be obedient means to be constantly attentive to this
active presence and to allow God, who is only love, to be the source
as well as the goal of all we think, say, and do.

Henri J. M. Nouwen

The gatekeeper opens the gate for him, and the sheep hear his voice.
He calls his own sheep by name and leads them out.
When he has brought out all his own, he goes ahead of them,
and the sheep follow him because they know his voice.
—JOHN 10:3–4

REFLECTION

Parents will often say of a child, "He doesn't listen," meaning that the child is
not obeying. From the child's point of view, obeying means doing what the
parent wants rather than the child's own will. But if the root of obedience is
listening, we have the opportunity to actively engage our hearts in hearing and
seeing the ways that God is present, going ahead of us in the experience of
caregiving. Wherever we go, we will find that God is already there.

- In what ways does God call your name as a caregiver and go ahead of you?
- In what environment do you feel most open to hear what God wants to say
  to you?

Great shepherd who sees and calls your sheep by name, reveal your
presence and love with bright surprises of the obedient life. Amen.

WOUNDED AND WEAK

We live in a world that suggests one person is strong and another person is weak, or some people have it together and others do not. And that those who are strong should help the weak. Now that's not what the gospel is speaking about. It belongs to the center of the gospel that God became vulnerable. That God stripped himself from power. That he didn't cling to his equality with God, but emptied himself and became a human being like we are. As a follower of Jesus, what I have to offer is first of all my own vulnerability. My own weakness, my own brokenness, my own wounds. My wounds can only be a source of healing for others if I care for my wounds, if I bandage them well with my willingness to create a fellowship of the weak and trust that there God's healing power will become visible.

Henri J. M. Nouwen

Let the same mind be in you that was in Christ Jesus,
who, though he was in the form of God,
   did not regard equality with God
   as something to be exploited,
but emptied himself,
   taking the form of a slave,
   being born in human likeness.
      —PHILIPPIANS 2:5–7

REFLECTION

As a caregiver you may feel that you have to be strong for the sake of the one you care for. When Jesus emptied himself of power and became human, as we are, he showed us that our weaknesses and vulnerabilities may be as much as a gift of caring as any experience of knowledge and competence. What we expect to see in the caregiving relationship may not be what God means for us to see. Reconsidering the balance of weak and strong may open our eyes.

- In what ways have you felt too weak to be a caregiver?
- How might accepting your own weakness change your relationship with the one you care for?

   God who offered vulnerability to a broken world, be the one who bandages wounds in a fellowship of the weak. Amen.

TO KNOW AND BE KNOWN

As Jesus ministers, so he wants us to minister. He told Peter to feed his sheep and care for them. He wants us to care not as "professionals" who know the clients' problems and take care of them but as vulnerable brothers and sisters who know and are known, who care and are cared for, who forgive and are being forgiven, who love and are being loved. Somehow we have come to believe that someone serves, someone else is being served, and be sure not to mix up the roles. We are not the healers, we are not the reconcilers, we are not the givers of life. We are sinful, broken, vulnerable people who need as much care as anyone we care for. The mystery of ministry is that we have been chosen to make our own limited and very conditional love the gateway for the unlimited and unconditional love of God.

Henri J. M. Nouwen

Jesus said to Simon Peter, "Simon son of John,
do you love me more than these?" He said to him,
"Yes, Lord; you know that I love you."
Jesus said to him, "Feed my lambs."
—JOHN 21:15

REFLECTION

Jesus chose Peter to lead the early church despite all of Peter's mistakes, for which he is famous. Jesus did not give the church a leader-shepherd who did not know what it was to feel weak or to have regrets. Few caregivers can rightly say they can think of nothing they wish they had done differently. We are vulnerable people caring for vulnerable people and receiving care from vulnerable people. This simple truth opens the gate for us to see each other and for love to flow.

- How do you respond to the idea that your vulnerability is a part of your caring?

- Do you open yourself to receiving the care of others, or do you resist it?

God who knows every vulnerability, by your unlimited love heal every limited resistance to know and be known for the deeper riches of caring. Amen.

FREE TO BE PRESENT

*Caregiving is a deeply ingrained human response to suffering. We want to
ease pain, to restore calm and peace to those in need. But caregiving takes a toll.
There is often a huge cost to the caregiver, and sometimes the care we give
springs not from a well of love and altruism but from a bitter sea of resentful
duty and obligation. It is hard to listen to others when the pains and troubles of
our own lives are clamoring for attention. But if we learn to listen to our own
needs and wants, that listening can free us to become truly present to the inner
deep and fragile beauty of those under our care. Even the most mundane
and repetitive caregiving tasks can become a means for us to grow.
With patience, with time, we can develop relationships of respect,
listening, presence, and truthfulness with those we care for.*

Henri J. M. Nouwen

I will both lie down and sleep in peace, for you alone,
O Lord, make me dwell in safety.
—PSALM 4:8

REFLECTION

Offering care easily becomes reduced to tasks—the sometimes unpleasant
activities. A bitter sea of resentful duty and obligation can roil with waves so
rough that we fear we will capsize. Then we feel guilty that caring is reduced
to tasks rather than perceiving it as a privilege of love. Our own health in the
caregiving process is vital to obediently listening to how God calls us to respond.
Something as simple as releasing the stress of caregiving long enough for a
good night's sleep can refresh both body and spirit.

- Using the imagery of a sea, how would you describe your relationship with
the person you care for?

- How might you receive care from others that would allow you respite
before bitterness sets in?

*God who sees every desire and need, make plain the path away from
the bitter sea and toward the patient presence of love. Amen.*

A GENTLE AND TENDER HAND

What does it mean to care? The word care *finds its roots in the Gothic* kara, *which means "lament." The basic meaning of care is to grieve, to experience sorrow, to cry out with. I am very much struck by this background of the word* care *because we tend to feel quite uncomfortable with an invitation to enter into someone's pain before doing something about it. Still, when we honestly ask ourselves which person in our lives means the most to us, we often find that it is those who, instead of giving much advice, solutions, or cures, have chosen rather to share our pain and touch our wounds with a gentle and tender hand. The friend who can be silent with us in a moment of despair, who can stay with us in an hour of grief, who can tolerate not-knowing, not-curing, not-healing—that is the friend who cares.*

Henri J. M. Nouwen

Moved with compassion, Jesus touched their eyes.
Immediately they regained their sight and followed him.
—MATTHEW 20:34

REFLECTION

Often the gospels describe Jesus healing individuals by saying that he touched them. Jesus is "moved with compassion" to touch, making touch a part of what it means to enter into the suffering of another. We are created both body and spirit, and compassionate care means in some way to touch both body and spirit. Often care requires physical touch, but touching the spirit is essential as well. Touch is assurance that we have been seen, whether giving or receiving care.

- What kind of touch, both bodily and spiritual, reassures you in your role as a caregiver?
- In what ways can you touch the spirit of the person you care for?

   God of compassion, may your touch be an example of entering another's lament with care even when there is no cure. Amen.

HEALING PRESENCE

To care means first of all to be present to each other. From experience you know that those who care for you become present to you. When they listen, they listen to you. When they speak, you know they speak to you. And when they ask questions, you know it is for your sake. Their presence is a healing presence because they accept you on your terms, and they encourage you to take your own life seriously and to trust your own vocation. Our tendency is to run away from the painful realities or to try to change them as soon as possible. But cure without care makes us into rulers, controllers, manipulators, and prevents a real community from taking shape. Cure without care makes us preoccupied with quick changes, impatient and unwilling to share each other's burden. And so cure can often become offending instead of liberating.

Henri J. M. Nouwen

Though I walk in the midst of trouble,
  you preserve me against the wrath of my enemies;
you stretch out your hand
  and your right hand delivers me.
  —PSALM 138:7

REFLECTION

The difference between *care* and *cure* colors how we relate to people in need of care, and how we open ourselves to care. In the gift of presence, we settle into *this* moment and allow it to change us. Scripture reminds us we do not walk alone in the midst of trouble, whether as one who gives care or one who receives it. Ultimately we find ourselves in both categories, and our path does not hurry past one or the other but bridges them both.

- In what ways have others been present to you in your vulnerable moments?
- How might understanding the meaning of presence change your caregiving?

God who is always present, reveal your caring touch.
Give us strength to be weak enough to see your light in the dark places. Amen.

WEEK 2

Our Greatest Gift

God's deep love is a revitalizing force lifting us when we have no more strength for the challenges of giving care We see God's love in and through one another.

THIS WEEK CONSIDER THIS QUESTION

Where do you most see God's love for you?

I **REALIZE VERY DEEPLY THAT LIFE** is hard for you with your family's illness and struggles. I'm glad to see, however, that your spirit is staying vital in the midst of it all and that you have the strength to keep some real freedom in your heart. I especially hope that you will be able to experience God's deep love for you and that this experience will allow you to remain compassionate for the many suffering people around you. Thank you again for writing. Be sure of my love.

GOING WHERE IT HURTS

*The word compassion is derived from the Latin words pati and cum,
which together mean "to suffer with." Compassion asks us to go where it hurts,
to enter places of pain, to share in brokenness, fear, confusion, and anguish.
Compassion challenges us to cry out with those in misery, to mourn with those
who are lonely, to weep with those in tears. Compassion requires us to be weak
with the weak, vulnerable with the vulnerable, and powerless with the powerless.
Compassion means full immersion in the condition of being human. Compassion
is not among our most natural responses. We are pain avoiders and we consider
anyone who feels attracted to suffering abnormal, or at least very unusual.*

Henri J. M. Nouwen

Sing for joy, O heavens, and exult, O earth;
break forth, O mountains, into singing!
For the Lord has comforted his people,
and will have compassion on his suffering ones.
—ISAIAH 49:13

REFLECTION

Is it possible to sing forth in the midst of suffering—whether our own or the
condition of a loved one? We may seek comfort because we are well aware of
our affliction. Or comfort may surprise us in an act of compassion and call us
out from behind our masks. Going where it hurts means we must be willing
to witness brokenness and not turn our heads. When we go to places of pain,
we carry with us the sure promise of God's comfort.

- What has been the most vulnerable experience in your caregiving story?
- Identify a gift of compassion that took your breath away. How did it change you?

*Lord of joy and Lord of song, break forth in your compassion.
Brighten sorrow with comfort only you can give. Amen.*

AN INNER DISPOSITION

Let us not underestimate how hard it is to be compassionate. Compassion is hard because it requires the inner disposition to go with others to the place where they are weak, vulnerable, lonely, and broken. But this is not our spontaneous response to suffering. What we desire most is to do away with suffering by fleeing from it or finding a quick cure for it. Our ability to enter into solidarity with those who suffer is our greatest gift.

Henri J. M. Nouwen

In all this I have given you an example that by such work we must support the weak, remembering the words of the Lord Jesus, for he himself said, "It is more blessed to give than to receive.'"

—ACTS 20:35

REFLECTION

The longer and more consistently we accept the call of compassion, the more we are in danger of wearing out, and the more we may be frustrated that we cannot offer a cure or a quick fix. Jesus said it is more blessed to give than to receive. This challenges us to offer the greater gift of enduring care, rather than quick cure. Our spontaneous impulse, which holds us outside the suffering, gives way to cultivating the inner disposition that allows us to discover the greatest gift.

- In what ways have you underestimated how hard it is to be compassionate?
- What do you desire most for the person you care for? And for yourself as a caregiver?

  Lord of compassion, make clear the path to go into the weak and broken places with the certainty that you are already there. Amen.

AMAZING GRACE

Moe's illnesses—Down's syndrome and Alzheimer's disease—showed the journey we all must make. But at the end of that journey, what do we finally see? Countless times Moe looked me in the eyes and said, "Amazing Grace." I was not always ready to sing the old song again, and often I would say, "Next time, Moe." Now Moe is gone, I keep hearing his persistent words—"Amazing Grace, Amazing Grace"—as God's way of announcing to me the mystery of Moe's life and of all people. We know that things will get harder as we get older and that the difference between people with a disability and those without a disability will become ever smaller. What are we ultimately growing toward? Are we growing into living reminders of that amazing grace that Moe always wanted to sing about?

Henri J. M. Nouwen

From his fullness we have all received, grace upon grace.
—JOHN 1:16

REFLECTION

In this simple verse, John reminds us of a truth that Moe seemed to know well. Jesus became human and lived among us. He knows full well our suffering because he has seen it and experienced it. The apostle turns our eyes to the gift of grace Jesus brought to us and emphasizes the fullness of Christ. "Grace upon grace" assures us that the grace of God will never be depleted. In the many moments of caregiving when we need amazing grace, it is available to us.

- Consider a time when you have experienced grace flowing in both directions between you and someone you care for.

- What experiences remind you of God's abundant and amazing grace offered to you?

> *Lord of all grace, may your movement be plain to see and multiplied in unexpected moments to fill empty spaces. Amen.*

THE CHOICE OF FAITH

The choice to see our own and other people's decreasing abilities as gateways to God's grace is a choice of faith. When John, the beloved disciple, looked up to Jesus and saw blood and water flowing from Jesus' pierced side, he saw something other than proof that all was over. He saw fulfillment of the prophecy that, "They will look up to the one whom they have pierced," a glimpse of God's victory over death. That is the choice of faith we make when we care for dying people with all the tenderness and gentleness that God's beloved children deserve. It's the choice that allows us to see the face of Jesus in the poor, the addicted, and those who live with AIDS and cancer. It's the choice of the human heart that has been touched by the Spirit of Jesus and is able to recognize that Spirit wherever people are dying.

Henri J. M. Nouwen

He who saw this has testified so that you also may believe.
His testimony is true, and he knows that he tells the truth.
—JOHN 19:35

REFLECTION

In John standing at the foot of the cross while Jesus died, we see someone who did not give way to obvious disappointment. The choice of faith allowed John to see God's movement and presence even under extreme circumstances. Caregiving can take us to extreme circumstances that demand inner resources. The choice of faith allows us know that God is there and to believe that God is able when we are unable. We have no victory of our own, but we trust in the truth of God's victory.

- How has your own faith been shaped by the experience of caregiving?
- Describe an experience when you have glimpsed God's victory over death.

*Lord of all—even death—help us to choose strong faith
and see your face lighting the dark places of doubt. Amen.*

A TASTE OF PAIN

God wants to know our condition fully and does not want to take away any pain
which he himself has not fully tasted. His compassion is anchored in the most
intimate solidarity. How do we know this is anything more than a beautiful idea?
How do we know that God is our God, and not a stranger, an outsider, a passerby?
We know this because in Jesus, God's compassion became visible to us. Jesus not
only said, "Be compassionate as your Father is compassionate," but he also was
the concrete embodiment of this divine compassion in our world.

Henri J. M. Nouwen

For he is our God,
   and we are the people of his pasture,
   and the sheep of his hand.
           —PSALM 95:7

REFLECTION

Caregiving is full of decisions. Sometimes the decisions are difficult because
the options are painful to imagine. Choosing compassion is what we desire,
but we too easily fail, and sometimes the caregiver needs care. The image of
being sheep in God's pasture reminds us that God's tenderness toward us is
faithful. Whether caregiver or care receiver, we belong to God, and God cares
for us. Only because of God's shepherding compassion in Jesus do we have a
glimmer of being compassionate to one another.

- How easy or difficult is it for you to be vulnerable about your experience
  of caregiving?
- In what ways does the image of God as a shepherd speak to your needs?

   God of compassion, may we know that you have tasted pain
   and willingly accept your shepherding care. Amen.

SAFE SPACE TO CARE

People living with disabilities are very vulnerable. They cannot hide their
weaknesses and therefore are easy victims of maltreatment and ridicule. But this
same vulnerability also allows them to bear ample fruit in the lives of those who
receive them. They are grateful people. They know they are dependent on others
and show this dependence every moment; but their smiles, embraces and kisses
are offered as spontaneous expressions of thanks. They know that all is pure gift
to be thankful for. They are people who need care. When they are locked up in
custodial institutions and treated as nobodies, they withdraw and cannot bear
fruit. They become overwhelmed by fears and close themselves to others. But
when they are given a safe space, with truly caring people whom they trust, they
soon become generous givers who are willing to offer their whole hearts.

Henri J. M. Nouwen

The Lord is my strength and my shield;
in him my heart trusts;
so I am helped, and my heart exults,
and with my song I give thanks to him.
—PSALM 28:7

REFLECTION

Caregivers are used to being the one to help, and perhaps the care receiver is
kind enough to express thanks. Gratitude itself is a gift that the care receiver
offers, and the caregiver has the opportunity to receive the gift with thankfulness
in return. Thankfulness then flows in both directions, bathing both caregiver
and care receiver in the strength of the Lord, on whom they both depend.
Thankfulness transforms the relationship to one of mutuality, rather than
one-sided dependence.

- How would you describe the role of thankfulness in your caregiving story?
- What fruit of thankfulness have you received from the person for whom
you care?

Lord of all gifts, may your fruit in the hearts of each one of your people multiply
generosity of spirit in our challenges and in our triumphs. Amen.

THOSE WHO MOURN

Sometimes we want to do every possible thing to change the circumstances of our life. We wish we were in another body, lived in another time, or had another mind! A cry can come out of our depths: Why do I have to be this person? I didn't ask for it, and I don't want it. But as we gradually come to befriend our own reality, to look with compassion at our own sorrows and joys, and as we are able to discover the unique potential of our way of being in the world, we can move beyond our protest, put the cup of our life to our lips, and drink it, slowly, carefully, but fully.

Henri J. M. Nouwen

"Blessed are those who mourn,
for they will be comforted."
—MATTHEW 5:4

REFLECTION

How can we learn to live in a way that does not grasp at what we have lost or are missing? How do we move through suffering rather than run away from it? The demands of caregiving, often while working or also looking after a family, mean that sometimes we do not slow down enough to express our own needs even to ourselves. If we do not name our losses, we also do not recognize the comfort that comes to those who mourn.

- What wounds does the experience of caregiving open in you? What do you mourn?
- How might your story of caregiving shape your understanding of God's ultimate purpose?

*Lord of comfort, hold the grasping hands of timid faith.
Manifest your blessing and make visible the good you can do
with the brokenness your people offer back to you. Amen.*

WEEK 3

An Invitation to Joy

Caregiving can be lonely and hard. It also changes us because we go into deep waters and return to the surface with something that can only come from the deep.

THIS WEEK CONSIDER THIS QUESTION

How is your story as a caregiver deepening your own experience of God?

Over the last few years I have been increasingly aware that true healing ministry takes place through the sharing of weakness. Mostly we are so afraid of our weaknesses that we hide them at all costs and thus make them unavailable to others but also to ourselves. And in this way we end up living double lives even against our own desires. One life in which we present ourselves to the world, to ourselves, and to God as a person who is in control and another life in which we feel insecure, doubtful, confused, and anxious, and totally out of control. The split between the two lives causes a lot of suffering.

I have become growingly aware of the importance to overcome the great chasm between these two lives and to become more and more aware that facing with others the reality of our existence can be the beginning of a truly free life. As long as I try to convince myself or others of my independence a lot of my energy is invested in building up my own false self. But once I am able to confess my most profound dependence on others and God, I can come in touch with my true self, and a real community can develop.

love
Henri.

JOY BEYOND SORROW

Dear Lord, give me eyes to see and ears to hear. I know there is a light in the darkness that makes everything new. I know there is new life in suffering that opens a new earth to me. I know there is a joy beyond sorrow that rejuvenates my heart. Yes, Lord, I know that you are, that you act, that you love, that you indeed are Light, Life, and Truth. People, work, plans, projects, ideas, meetings, buildings, paintings, music and literature all can only give me real joy and peace when I can see and hear them as reflections of your presence, your glory, your kingdom. Let me see and hear what is real, and let me have the courage to keep unmasking endless unrealities, which disturb my life every day. Now I see only in a mirror, but one day, O Lord, I hope to see you face to face. Amen.

Henri J. M. Nouwen

You have turned my mourning into dancing;
    you have taken off my sackcloth
    and clothed me with joy,
so that my soul may praise you and not be silent.
    O Lord my God, I will give thanks to you forever.
        —PSALM 30:11–12

REFLECTION

How easy it is to narrow our vision when we are wrapped in the concerns of caregiving. Perhaps even our prayers revolve around caregiving. Is it possible to see a season of caregiving in the context of life that goes on around us? Doing so requires a lens of expectation of seeing God active and moving in all the parts of our stories. The cares and concerns of caregiving are balanced by the rejuvenating assurance of God's presence.

- In what ways has your caregiving vision narrowed? What would you like to see instead?

- What would be your own prayer for joy beyond sorrow?

    *O God, give us expectant hearts seeking assurance of your presence.
    Be the light in the darkness that makes all things new. Amen.*

JOY REVEALS JOY

*I realize that I am not used to the image of God throwing a big party. It seems
to contradict the solemnity and seriousness I have always attached to God.
But when I think about the ways in which Jesus describes God's kingdom, a joyful
banquet is often at its center. Every moment of each day I have the chance to
choose between cynicism and joy. Every thought I have can be cynical or joyful.
Every word I speak can be cynical or joyful. Every action can be cynical or joyful.
Increasingly I am aware of all these possible choices, and increasingly I discover
that every choice for joy in turn reveals more joy and offers more reason
to make life a true celebration in the house of the Father.*

Henri J. M. Nouwen

"But the father said to his slaves ... 'let us eat and celebrate;
for this son of mine was dead and is alive again; he was
lost and is found!' And they began to celebrate."
—LUKE 15:22–24

REFLECTION

In the story of the prodigal son, the older brother feels cheated. Why should his
errant little brother be welcomed home? We might say he is still cynical and
cannot see his way to joy. His father, though, is fully given over to joy. Cynicism
can become a habit; everything is suspect, nothing is trustworthy. The first
glimmer of joy in caregiving can change not only the habit of cynicism but the
manner in which we offer the gift of care. Joy reveals more joy.

- On the spectrum of cynicism and joy, where would you place yourself?
- Think about a moment of joy in your caregiving story. What further joy
  did that moment reveal?

> *O God, joy is the right choice, yet falling back into cynicism
> can be so much easier. Through your gift of joy, prepare
> the feast and beckon the weary and wounded. Amen.*

A GIFT OFFERED

Joy and gratitude are the qualities of heart by which we recognize those who are committed to a life of service in the path of Jesus Christ. We see this in families where parents and children are attentive to one another's needs and spend time together despite many outside pressures. We see it in those who always have room for a stranger, an extra plate for a visitor, time for someone in need. We see it in the many men and women who offer money, time and energy for those who are hungry, in prison, sick or dying. Just as a mother does not need to be rewarded for the attention she pays to her child, because her child is her joy, so those who serve their neighbor will find their reward in the people whom they serve.

Henri J. M. Nouwen

Can a woman forget her nursing child,
   or show no compassion for the child of her womb?
Even these may forget,
   yet I will not forget you.
See, I have inscribed you on the palms of my hands;
   your walls are continually before me.
          —ISAIAH 49:15–16

REFLECTION

Often caregiving feels like a role thrust upon us by circumstances. It's the "right" thing to do, but we may wish—at least some of the time—for an alternative. The image of a woman who cannot forget her child is apt because it is wrapped in love that does not let go. Isaiah's words assure us that this is how God sees us. This place of secure belonging is the beginning of joy and gratitude that shapes our service.

- How would you describe the relationship between joy, gratitude, and caregiving?
- What is your story of being forgotten amid the service of caregiving?

   *O God, open wide your hands to show that you are always near
   and you do not forget those whom you have called. Amen.*

A SIMPLE PRESENCE

Joy is hidden in compassion. The word compassion *literally means "to suffer with." It seems quite unlikely that suffering with another person would bring joy. Yet being with a person in pain, offering simple presence to someone in despair, sharing with a friend times of confusion and uncertainty ... such experiences can bring us deep joy. Not happiness, not excitement, not great satisfaction, but the quiet joy of being there for someone else and living in deep solidarity with our brothers and sisters in this human family. Often there is a solidarity in weakness, in brokenness, in woundedness, but it leads to the center of joy, which is sharing our humanity with others.*

Henri J. M. Nouwen

Blessed be the God and Father of our Lord Jesus Christ, the Father of mercies and the God of all consolation, who consoles us in all our affliction, so that we may be able to console those who are in any affliction with the consolation with which we ourselves are consoled by God. For just as the sufferings of Christ are abundant for us, so also our consolation is abundant through Christ.
—2 CORINTHIANS 1:3–5

REFLECTION

Suffering and consolation can be such visceral experiences! Suffering *with* someone, not as an onlooker only but in true solidarity, changes us. Paul's words to the Corinthians remind us that because God has consoled us, we are able to console others. And consolation is *abundant*. There is no lack when God is the source. In the solidarity of compassion, we find the joy that comes from God, and despite the circumstances we are changed in the way we welcome and serve others.

- What gets in the way of our standing in solidarity and sharing humanity?

- How has an experience of being consoled by God changed your caregiving story?

   O God, all compassion and consolation come from you. When hearts of joy in service turn to your face, you are always there. Amen.

A JOY IN COMMUNITY

In my own community, with many men and women living with disabilities,
the greatest source of suffering is not the disability itself, but the accompanying
feelings of being useless, worthless, unappreciated and unloved. It is much easier
to accept the inability to speak, walk or feed oneself than it is to accept the inability
to be of special value to another person. We human beings can suffer immense
deprivations with great steadfastness, but when we sense that we no longer have
anything to offer to anyone, we quickly lose our grip on our life. Instinctively
we know that the joy of life comes from the ways in which we live together and
that the pain of life comes from the many ways we fail to do that well.

Henri J. M. Nouwen

If one member suffers, all suffer together with it; if one
member is honored, all rejoice together with it. Now you
are the body of Christ and individually members of it.
—1 CORINTHIANS 12:26–27

REFLECTION

Depending on the needs of the person you care for, you may well recognize the
thought that the sense of having nothing to offer causes great suffering. You
may even feel that *you* have nothing left to offer the person you care for. Be
careful not to measure value by what you or another person can do independently,
but rather affirm your connection with others simply because we are all human
beings created and loved by God. In caring rather than curing, we share both
pain and joy.

- In what ways have you seen living well with others to be a source of joy?
- How do you get back on track when you feel you have failed to live well
  with the person you care for?

O God, suffering together and rejoicing together form your people
to live well in your service together. Make yourself known in the
moments, no matter what they bring. Amen.

A LASTING GRACE

It is good to visit people who are sick, dying, shut in, disabled, or lonely. But it is also important not to feel guilty when our visits have to be cut short or can only happen occasionally. Often we are so apologetic about our limitations that our apologies prevent us from really being with the other when we are there. A short time fully present to a sick person is much better than a long time with many explanations of why we are too busy to come more often. If we are able to be fully present when we are with them, our absence too will bear many fruits. Our friends will say, "He visited me" or "She visited me" and discover in our absence the lasting grace of our presence.

Henri J. M. Nouwen

See what love the Father has given us, that we should be called children of God; and that is what we are ... Beloved, we are God's children now.

—1 JOHN 3:1–2

REFLECTION

It is not always easy to know what to say to someone who is suffering, whether physically, emotionally, spiritually, or all three. Perhaps we change the subject or offer a trite encouragement. Going deeper means being willing to see through the eyes of another those moments of uncertainty of value or even despair. We don't want to minimize what another person feels, but if we can gently be reminders of God's full acceptance of us as beloved children, we will have served well.

- How much do you struggle to be seen, praised, or admired in your caregiving story?
- Meditate on an experience you've had of feeling embraced by God as a child of God.

> *O God, we are beloved because you call us so. Help us in our weakness when we forget to whom we belong. Amen.*

CHILDREN OF THE LIGHT

The experience of God's acceptance frees us from our needy self and thus creates new space in which we can pay selfless attention to others. This new freedom in Christ allows us to move in the world uninhibited by our compulsions and to act creatively even when we are laughed at and rejected. Only a life of ongoing, intimate communion with God can reveal to us our true selfhood; only such a life can set us free to act, according to the truth, and not according to our need for the spectacular. This is far from easy. A serious and persevering discipline of solitude, silence and prayer is demanded Such a discipline will not reward us with the outer glitter of success, but with the inner light which enlightens our whole being and which allows us to be free and uninhibited witnesses of God's presence in our lives.

Henri J. M. Nouwen

Beloved, let us love one another, because love is from God; everyone who loves is born of God and knows God. ... We love because he first loved us.
—1 JOHN 4:7, 19

REFLECTION

If we're honest, some of us shut down at the suggestion of "ongoing intimate communion with God." We don't know how to do that! Perhaps we need to begin with just one single minute of stillness and deep breathing, meditating on the transforming love of God. Over time, one minute might grow into five or ten or thirty. We each come in our own way and in our own time to experience God's full acceptance of us and the ways in which it will free us to serve.

- Look back over the time you've been a caregiver. How has the story changed you?

- In what ways has a spiritual inner light freed you to embrace caregiving more fully?

O God, your great love and light bind all things together, even as you have poured out your love for the sake of those you call to yourself. Help us to joyfully accept your gift. Amen.

WEEK 4

A Prayer for Caring

Caregiving feels solitary. We look out from our own lives and see so many people who seem not to experience what we feel. But we are not alone. Christ and caring friends are our companions.

THIS WEEK CONSIDER THIS QUESTION

How do you see Christ in the people who are part of your day?

IT IS SO IMPORTANT FOR YOU TO have a place where you can go to pray, be quiet, and meet some very caring people. When you have such a place where your heart can be nurtured it will also be easier to see Christ. Only when Christ really is alive in your heart can you recognize him in your neighbor, because it is Christ in you who calls forth the Christ in the other. I really feel it is very important for you to have a regular discipline of prayer and spiritual reading. That and some caring friends will allow you to live through these very painful and difficult years and will prevent your heart from becoming bitter and resentful. Be sure that I always pray for you and both your sons.

love

Henri.

THE PROMISED SPIRIT

*The Holy Spirit whom Jesus promised to his followers is the great gift of God.
Without the Spirit of Jesus we can do nothing, but in and through his Spirit we can
live free, joyful and courageous lives. We cannot pray, but the Spirit of Christ can
pray in us. We cannot create peace and joy, but the Spirit of Christ can fill us with
a peace and joy which is not of this world. We cannot break through the many
barriers which divide races, sexes and nations, but the Spirit of Christ unites all
people in the all-embracing love of God. The Spirit of Christ burns away our many
fears and anxieties, and sets us free to move wherever we are sent.*

Henri J. M. Nouwen

Likewise the Spirit helps us in our weakness; for we do not
know how to pray as we ought, but that very Spirit intercedes
with sighs too deep for words. And God, who searches the heart,
knows what is the mind of the Spirit, because the Spirit
intercedes for the saints according to the will of God.
—ROMANS 8:26–27

REFLECTION

Life reminds us every day what we cannot do. In fact, we may feel that the harder
we try, the less we succeed with our good intentions. We want to pray more,
love more, serve more, care more, give more. Yet what we desire remains out of
reach. We live in weakness, but Christ is our strength. We do not strive on our
own. Rather, we step into what the Spirit of Christ is doing and find our place
there. Then we will be free.

- Reflect on something you have had to rely on the Spirit of Christ for.
- In what ways do you need to be set free to move where you are sent as a
  caregiver?

*O Lord, your Spirit is freedom from striving and
fracturing. May your Spirit lead the way into freedom
of peace and joy that is not of this world. Amen.*

A CRY FOR MERCY

For most of us it is hard to spend a useless hour with God. It is hard precisely because by facing God alone we are also facing our own inner chaos. We come in direct confrontation with our restlessness, anxieties, and resentments, unresolved tensions, hidden animosities, and long-standing frustrations. Our spontaneous reaction to all this is to run away and get busy again. It is the painful stripping away of the old self, this falling away from all our old support system, that enables us to cry out for the unconditional mercy of God. When we do not run away in fear, but patiently stay with our struggles, the outer space of solitude gradually becomes an inner space, a space in our heart where we come to know the presence of the Spirit who has already been given to us.

Henri J. M. Nouwen

By the tender mercy of our God,
the dawn from on high will break upon us.
—LUKE 1:78

REFLECTION

A "useless hour with God." For such an encounter we must let our guards down. Everything we strive to protect and accomplish must be let go so that we come to God with our full attention and openness of heart. God is not afraid of the mess that we hesitate to show. When we want to hurry back to be in control, God calls us closer with tender mercy that allows us to see our circumstances in new light.

- How would you describe your own inner chaos?

- Where is one place where you can go to seek an outer space of solitude?

Our God, unclasp the fingers that hold inner chaos too close. Shed your light on the darkness. Prepare wrestling hearts to meet your tender mercy. Amen.

"ABBA, FATHER"

The discipline of the heart is the discipline by which we create the inner space in which the Spirit of God can cry out in us, "Abba, Father." Thus through the discipline of the heart we reach the heart of God. When we come to hear the heartbeat of God in the intimacy of our prayer, we realize that God's heart embraces all the sufferings of the world. We come to see that through Jesus Christ these burdens have become a light burden which we are invited to carry. Prayer always leads to the heart of God and the heart of the human struggle at the same time. It is in the heart of God that we come to understand the true nature of human suffering and come to know our mission to alleviate this suffering, not in our name but in the name of one who suffered and through his suffering overcame all evil.

Henri J. M. Nouwen

For all who are led by the Spirit of God are children of God. For you did not receive a spirit of slavery to fall back into fear, but you have received a spirit of adoption. When we cry, "Abba! Father!" it is that very Spirit bearing witness with our spirit.
—ROMANS 8:14–16

REFLECTION

We are beloved children of God, yet we sometimes hesitate to be intimate with God, ready to uncover our vulnerabilities and exchange our self-doubt for God's embrace. We understand struggling and suffering. We have less understanding that even through struggling and suffering God forms our hearts to know his more freely. When we cry out in the midst of a burden, we feel it lifted by Jesus himself. When we offer care, we offer the heart and love of God to another person. We are not alone.

- How do you feel about the word *discipline* in your relationship with God?
- How can prayer coexist with struggle and suffering?

Our God, your heart beats for all creation. Your arms are open wide to receive the doubter and the fearful. Thank you that you never hide your heart from your children. Amen.

GOD OF THE LIVING

*Dear Lord, by the power that went out from you a woman was healed of an illness
no doctor had been able to cure and a young girl was called to life. You revealed
that God is the God of life in whom no death can be found. Touch our
death-oriented world and call forth new life. Bring life, joy and new vitality
to those who are walking in the shadow of death, to those who are depressed
and in despair, to those who are resentful and violent. Do not let your people be
conquered by these dark forces, but let your life-giving power enter their bodies,
hearts and minds, and let them recognize you as the Son of God who is not
a God of the dead but of the living. Amen.*

Henri J. M. Nouwen

The women were terrified and bowed their faces to the ground,
but the men said to them, "Why do you look for the living
among the dead? He is not here, but has risen."
—LUKE 24:5

REFLECTION

The power of death is at work not only in the failing of our physical bodies but
in emotions and spirits and relationships and discouragement and doubt. It is
no stretch of the imagination to see the world as a place consumed by death.
But in the healing miracles of Jesus and ultimately in the resurrection, we see
God's alternative—life! Abundant life flows from the source of all life. As
caregivers, when we choose this lens we see hope and meaning.

- When have you expected to see death and instead discovered life?
- Name a person or experience that helps the life of God flow into you.

*Our God, your life-giving power is greater than any form of loss.
May this glad understanding raise up the down-in-heart to a
new vitality of love and service for you. Amen.*

THE ABUNDANCE OF GOD'S GIFTS

Fear and anxiety never totally leave us. But slowly they lose their domination as a deeper and more central experience begins to present itself. It is the experience of gratitude. Gratitude is the awareness that life in all its manifestations is a gift for which we want to give thanks. The closer we come to God in prayer, the more we become aware of the abundance of God's gifts to us. We may even discover the presence of these gifts in the midst of our pains and sorrows. The mystery of the spiritual life is that many of the events, people and situations that for a long time seemed to inhibit our way to God become ways of our being united more deeply with him. What seemed a hindrance proves to be a gift. Thus gratitude becomes a quality of our hearts that allows us to live joyfully and peacefully even though our struggles continue.

Henri J. M. Nouwen

And let the peace of Christ rule in your hearts, to which
indeed you were called in the one body. And be thankful.
—COLOSSIANS 3:15

REFLECTION

Gratitude is a powerful force—in renewing human relationships, in drawing us closer to God, in helping us see the struggles of life and caregiving in new light. And not only do we see differently, we enter more fully into our stories and expect that God will be present in our sorrows. From our limited human experience, peace may be external and fleeting—a time without too many trials—but from God's perspective, peace flows out of knowing God more deeply.

- Name some fears and anxieties that have never totally left you. What effect have they had?

- If you had a great level of inner peace, how might that change your caregiving story?

Our God, a joyous variety of life reveals the unlimited ways to know you and to bask in your healing love with grateful hearts. Amen.

"COME TO ME"

To pray is to unite ourselves with Jesus and lift up the whole world through him to God in a cry of forgiveness, reconciliation, healing and mercy. To pray, therefore, is to connect whatever human pain or struggle we encounter—whether starvation, torture, displacement of peoples, or any form of physical or mental anguish—with the gentle and human heart of Jesus. Prayer is leading every sorrow to the source of all healing; it is letting the warmth of Jesus' love melt the cold anger of resentment; it is opening a space where joy replaces sadness, mercy supplants bitterness, love displaces fear, gentleness and care overcome hatred and indifference. But most of all prayer is the way to become and remain part of Jesus' mission to draw all people to the intimacy of God's love.

Henri J. M. Nouwen

"Come to me, all you that are weary and are carrying heavy burdens, and I will give you rest. Take my yoke upon you, and learn from me; for I am gentle and humble in heart, and you will find rest for your souls. For my yoke is easy, and my burden is light."

—MATTHEW 11:28–30

REFLECTION

Sorrow invades our spirits—and eventually our actions. Resentment and anxiety may be birthed by sorrow that weighs on us as a heavy burden. And though we may know that prayer draws us closer to God, we may be so burdened that we do not have strength to pray. Even in those times, we are not alone. Jesus says, "Come to me." That includes the weariness of caregiving. Rest and healing await us in the heart of Jesus.

- What obstacles might you face in bringing your own sorrow to a place of healing?

- How might your prayers draw the person you care for into the intimacy of God's love?

Our God, your love provides a restful place to heal and be strengthened. May stubbornness fade into the security that no burden is too great to give to you. Amen.

FROM ETERNITY TO ETERNITY

*What can we say about God's love? We can say that God's love is unconditional.
God does not say, "I love you if..." There are no ifs in God's heart. God's love for us
does not depend on what we do or say, on our looks or intelligence on our success
or our popularity. God's love for us existed before we were born and will exist
after we die. God's love exists from eternity to eternity. Does that mean God does
not care what we do or say? No, because God's love wouldn't be real if God didn't
care. To love without condition does not mean to love without concern.
God desires to enter into relationship with us and wants us to love God in return.
Let's dare to enter into an intimate relationship with God without fear,
trusting that we will receive love and always more love.*

Henri J. M. Nouwen

For I am convinced that neither death, nor life, nor angels, nor
rulers, nor things present, nor things to come, nor powers, nor
height, nor depth, nor anything else in all creation, will be able to
separate us from the love of God in Christ Jesus our Lord.
—ROMANS 8:38–39

REFLECTION

Love that extends "from eternity to eternity" is difficult to comprehend. It asks
us to see beyond our immediate circumstances in a cause-and-effect existence
to a transcending presence. Something so far beyond ourselves may tempt us
to believe God does not care about our circumstances. God does care—enough
to reach across eternity and touch our hearts when we feel alone or distressed.
Though we cannot measure eternity, we can know that nothing separates us
from the love of God.

- What emotions do you feel when you hear the phrase "from eternity
  to eternity"?
- What words might you add to the list in Romans 8 of forces that cannot
  separate you from God's love?

  *Our God, hearts hunger for greater assurance in the hard moments.
  "Give us this day our daily bread"—and the security of eternity. Amen.*

WEEK 5

The Voice of Love

Caregiving is consuming—of time, money, emotions. And often we feel an unspoken loss of what might have been as we wrestle with what is.

THIS WEEK CONSIDER THIS QUESTION

Amid the demands of caregiving, how is preserving a healthy sense of self rooted in what it means to be God's beloved?

BE SURE NOT TO LOSE YOUR life in the lives of your husband and your son. Their lives are best served when you can claim your own life as unique and different from theirs. I know this is easy to write, but I write it to encourage you to take some time for yourself, to read, to pray, to go out with friends, to enjoy nature, to listen to music. Your life is unique in God's eyes just as your son's and your husband's life. Somehow I feel that your suffering will bear many fruits, even though they are not visible yet.

love
Henri

THE GOD WHO COMES

I wonder if depression in the spiritual life does not mean that we have forgotten that prayer is grace. The deep realization that all the fruits of the spiritual life are gifts from God should make us smile, and liberate us from any deadly seriousness. We can close our eyes as tightly as we can, and clasp our hands as firmly as possible, but God speaks only when he wants to speak. When we realize this, our pressing, pushing and pulling become quite amusing. After having done everything to make some space for God, it is still God who comes on his own initiative. But we have the promise of his love. So our life can rightly be a waiting in expectation, but waiting patiently and with a smile. Then indeed we shall be really surprised and full of joy when he comes.

Henri J. M. Nouwen

But this I call to mind,
   and therefore I have hope:
The steadfast love of the Lord never ceases,
   his mercies never come to an end;
they are new every morning;
   great is your faithfulness.
      —LAMENTATIONS 3:21–23

REFLECTION

What do we pray for? Certainty that we are doing the right thing? A positive turn in our health or the health of someone we care for? Answers to deep questions about the experience of caregiving? Often our prayers are full of requests that God will act. If prayer is grace, and God comes to us on divine initiative, perhaps our deepest prayer is not for God's action, but for God's presence. Our spiritual life makes us ready to welcome God into our stories.

- Has depression in the spiritual life manifested in your caregiving story?
- What is the most meaningful way that you make space to welcome God?

God who comes, show afresh that you lighten spirits of those who seek you because your divine initiative wraps your people in your presence and the promise of hope. Amen.

THE TRUE SELF

My true self is rooted in the One who calls me the beloved, and who says to me,
"I love you with an everlasting love. I have loved you before you were born.
And I love you after you have died. I am embracing you from all eternity to all
eternity. I am saying I love you, I love you, I love you, with an everlasting love.
I am just giving you a few years to live to be able to say in return, 'I love you too.'"
That is what life is about spiritually.

Henri J. M. Nouwen

For the wind passes over it, and it is gone,
　and its place knows it no more.
But the steadfast love of the Lord is from
　everlasting to everlasting
　on those who fear him,
　and his righteousness to children's children.
　　　　—PSALM 103:16–17

REFLECTION

Life is an exchange of love that begins with God. Even in the daily grind of caregiving, God calls us—both caregiver and care receiver—"beloved." We are able to join the story of God's love in our love for those for whom we care. And in this we find hope, not despair; understanding, not abandonment; encouragement, not anguish. God's love is wide enough to hear all our cries and steady enough to answer them with God's own heart.

- What three words would you use to describe your true self?

- What forces do you feel pulling against your true self?

God who loves, grant a glimpse of eternity that your arms hold
in wait for your beloveds. May we know it better and learn to both receive
and return your love. Amen.

CHOSEN BY GOD

The great spiritual battle begins—and never ends—with the reclaiming of our chosenness. Long before any human being saw us, we are seen by God's loving eyes. Long before anyone has heard us cry or laugh, we are heard by our God who is all ears for us. Long before any person spoke to us in this world, we are spoken to by the voice of eternal love. Our preciousness, uniqueness, and individuality are not given to us by those who meet us in clock-time—our brief chronological existence—but by the One who has chosen us with an everlasting love, a love that existed from all eternity and will last through all eternity.

Henri J. M. Nouwen

And a voice from heaven said, "This is my Son,
the Beloved, with whom I am well pleased."
—MATTHEW 3:17

REFLECTION

At the beginning of his public ministry, Jesus was baptized. As he came out of the water, God called Jesus "the Beloved." God offers to us the same experience of belonging and belovedness. As we take our cue from Jesus, we find the path of caregiving lit with the twin lights of listening to God and offering obedience in our own ministries, including caregiving in a way that invites those we care for into God's belovedness.

- Do you think of your relationship with God based on your choosing God or God's choosing you?

- In what ways have your heard God calling you beloved?

God who chooses us, give grace to grasp the gift of being loved by you. Show the quiet places that illumine the path of obedience. Amen.

THE LIGHT WE CARRY

Often we want to be able to see into the future. We say, "How will next year be for me? Where will I be five or ten years from now?" There are no answers to these questions. Mostly we have just enough light to see the next step: what we have to do in the coming hour or the following day. The art of living is to enjoy what we can see and not complain about what remains in the dark. When we are able to take the next step with the trust that we will have enough light for the step that follows, we can walk through life with joy and be surprised at how far we go.

Let's rejoice in the little light we carry and not ask for the great beam of light that would take all shadows away.

Henri J. M. Nouwen

Again Jesus spoke to them, saying, "I am the light of the world. Whoever follows me will never walk in darkness but will have the light of life."
—JOHN 8:12

REFLECTION

Caregiving comes in various forms. Some are brief seasons we travel through and others seemingly unending stretches. Sometimes we see the light at the end of the tunnel, and other times we have only light for the step just ahead. Whether we try to see ahead five steps or five years, we take comfort in Jesus' words that he is the light. We do not walk in darkness, and we do not walk alone.

- What aspects of your caregiving story do you enjoy?

- What aspects tempt you to complain about what remains in the dark?

God who lights the way, stir up joyfulness because of your presence on the journey and grant the gift of confidence to follow where you lead. Amen.

THE SELF-PORTRAIT

There can hardly be a better image of caring than that of the artist who brings new life to people by an honest and fearless self-portrait. Rembrandt painted his sixty-five self-portraits not just as "a model for studies in expression" but as "a search for the spiritual through the channel of the innermost personality."* Rembrandt felt that he had to enter into his own self, into his dark cellars as well as into his light rooms if he really wanted to penetrate the mystery of the human interior. While growing in age he was more able to touch the core of the human experience, in which individuals in their misery can recognize themselves and find "courage and new youth." We will never be able to really care if we are not willing to paint and repaint constantly our self-portrait as a service to those who are searching for some light in the midst of darkness.

Henri J. M. Nouwen

Then God said, "Let there be light"; and there was light. And God saw that the light was good; and God separated the light from the darkness.
—GENESIS 1:3–4

REFLECTION

It would seem that the older Rembrandt grew, the better he understood himself. No matter our age, we can look back and recognize the experiences that shaped our story. Sometimes this calls for courage. Our older selves might like to give our younger selves some advice, but we are never too old to be looking for the light that God brings into our dark spaces as we understand more and more that, above all, we are God's beloved.

- What encouragement from your caregiving story might help someone else see light?
- If you drew sixty-five self-portraits, how do you think they might change over the course of your caregiving story?

God who separates light from darkness, may awareness grow that your light is good, and that welcoming you into dark spaces also gives strength to stand in your healing light. Amen.

**Quoted portions are from* Rembrandt Paintings *by Horst Gerson (New York: Reynal and Company, 1968), p. 460.*

ACTIVE EXPECTATION

Hope is something other than optimism. Hope is not based on statistics. Hope is based on the promise of God who entered into a human covenant with his people and pledged unwavering faithfulness. There is hope for history not because of bright human predictions we can come up with—there are none anyhow— but because our God is a God who so loved his people that he sent his only Son to become fully part of history, and to guide it not to destruction but to fulfillment.

Henri J. M. Nouwen

On that day the deaf shall hear
   the words of a scroll,
and out of their gloom and darkness
   the eyes of the blind shall see.
The meek shall obtain fresh joy in the Lord,
   and the neediest people shall exult in the
   Holy One of Israel.
                    —ISAIAH 29:18–19

REFLECTION

Do we give up hope, or do we give up our need to control? Caregiving is full of circumstances we cannot control. The vigilance of caregiving can be wearying. Because we have faith, we know that even the things we cannot control are in the loving hands of God. Isaiah's words give us the assurance of God's redemptive presence. We let go of our grip, and our fatigue, because we know those we love are also God's beloved.

- On a spectrum of feeling like nothing you do matters at one end and hoping in God's love at the other, where would you put yourself today?

- How might the love of God move you to a place of refreshment?

God who gives all life, grant courage to look deeply and find you in the eyes of all we meet. Even at a point of greatest need, you will be there. Amen.

HOPE AND JOY IN FAITH

Trust is the basis of life. Without trust no human being can live. Trapeze artists offer a beautiful image of this. Flyers have to trust their catchers. They can do the most spectacular doubles, triples, and quadruples, but what finally makes their performances spectacular are the catchers who are there for them at the right time in the right place Much of our lives is flying. It is wonderful to fly in the air free as a bird, but when God isn't there to catch us, all our flying comes to nothing Let's trust the Great Catcher.

Henri J. M. Nouwen

"I have said this to you, so that in me you may have peace. In the world you face persecution. But take courage; I have conquered the world!"
—JOHN 16:33

REFLECTION

Hope. Joy. Faith. Love. Trust. Sometimes we feel these words, and sometimes we don't. The renewal trust brings is familiar, yet we still find ourselves swinging between faith and skepticism—and wishing we had more control over things and could be sure of positive outcomes. Jesus' words in John 16:33 remind us that we do not take on the world in our own strength. Jesus has conquered the world, and this truth—this ultimate trust—is what gives us courage to continue in our callings.

- In what circumstances have you seen yourself resist letting go to trust God?
- In what circumstances have you seen the renewal that greater trust brings?

God who gives courage, you have indeed conquered the world. Grant to your beloved children increased faith, deepened trust, multiplied joy, and shining hope in your love. Amen.

WEEK 6

Rise to New Life

Caregiving is a calling born of love. It can be isolating and sacrificial and wearying, yet love remains and sustains. When we know deeply the love of God, we see the beloved in others.

THIS WEEK CONSIDER THIS QUESTION

What has been the greatest triumph of love in your story?

AS YOU MAY ALREADY KNOW, I have been pastor of the L'Arche Daybreak community since 1986. When I left the academic world, I really did not know what living and working with people with mental disabilities would mean. I can now truly tell you that my life at Daybreak has been an enormous joy and growth for me, and has filled me with new hope and new joy. I have become more and more aware that Jesus did not say, "Blessed are those who care for the poor," but "Blessed are the poor." The people in our community who are called "disabled" or "handicapped" are the ones who, in fact, carry a very unique blessing with them for the healing and renewal of the Spirit.

love

Henri

THE CHOICE TO CARE WELL

*To care well for the dying we must trust that these people are loved as much as we
are; we must trust that their dying and death deepen their solidarity with the
human family, and we must guide them in becoming part of the communion of
saints; and finally we must trust that their death, just as ours, will make their lives
fruitful for generations to come. We must encourage them to let go of their fears
and to hope beyond the boundaries of death. We are constantly tempted to think
that we have nothing or little to offer our fellow human beings. Their despair
frightens us. It often seems better not to come close than to come close without
being able to change anything. Whenever we claim our gift of care and choose
to embrace not only our own mortality, but also other people's,
we can become a true source of healing and hope.*

Henri J. M. Nouwen

The Lord bless you and keep you;
the Lord make his face to shine upon you,
   and be gracious to you;
the Lord lift up his countenance upon you,
   and give you peace.
   —NUMBERS 6:24–26

REFLECTION

Caregiving is in the here and now, where we must advocate with a steady heart,
sometimes cajole, and always bring tenderness to our caregiving tasks. We may
feel bogged down in the demands of the moment, but skin-to-skin and eye-to-
eye connection with those we care for holds great meaning. Let those liminal
moments raise our spirits to hope beyond the boundaries of death and stare
into the brightness of God's countenance shining upon us.

- Have you known despair that frightens you? What truth did you grasp to
  find your way to hope?

- No matter how long you've been caregiving, in what ways do you choose
  to claim your gift of care?

*God who gives peace, call each one by name so that we'll lift our heads to listen.
Be in our moments, our days, our years with your steadfast love. Amen.*

THE CHOICE TO DIE WELL

We will all die one day. That is one of the few things we can be sure of. But will we die well? That is less certain. Dying well means dying for others, making our lives fruitful for those we leave behind. The big question therefore is not, "What can I still do in the years I have left to live?" but "How can I prepare myself for my death so my life can continue to bear fruit in the generations that will follow me?" Jesus died well because through dying he sent his Spirit of Love to his friends, who with that Holy Spirit could live better lives. Can we also send the Spirit of Love to our friends when we leave them? Or are we too worried about what we can still do?

Dying can become our greatest gift if we prepare ourselves to die well.

Henri J. M. Nouwen

"I came that they may have life, and have it abundantly."
—JOHN 10:10

REFLECTION

Many caregivers know the path of walking with a loved one in the last weeks and days of life. As we offer a healing presence to someone who may soon see the face of Jesus, we ask ourselves what *we* are leaving to those who follow behind us. A good way to examine the fruit we will leave is to name the fruit offered to us by those we care for now. Seeing the abundance of God's grace even in death will form our hearts in gratitude.

- As you give care, what are your thoughts about a time when you might need care?

- What have you learned about the abundant life through your story of caregiving?

    God who gives your Spirit, fill the empty places in us so that each life takes on your goodness in fruit that nourishes others. Amen.

LOVE EVERLASTING

The resurrection does not solve our problems about dying and death. It is not the happy ending to our life's struggle, nor is it the big surprise that God has kept in store for us. No, the resurrection is the expression of God's faithfulness to Jesus and to all God's children. Through the resurrection God has said to Jesus, "You are indeed my beloved Son and my love is everlasting." And to us God has said, "You indeed are my beloved children and my love is everlasting." The resurrection is God's way of revealing to us that nothing that belongs to God will ever go to waste. What belongs to God will never get lost—not even our mortal bodies.

Henri J. M. Nouwen

For the mountains may depart
and the hills be removed,
but my steadfast love shall not depart from you,
and my covenant of peace shall not be removed,
says the Lord, who has compassion on you.
—ISAIAH 54:10

REFLECTION

Even though we place our trust in Christ's sacrificial death and triumphal resurrection, we still know suffering and death. We see the deterioration of body and mind and yearn for the day when there will be no more crying. But God's word for us through Jesus' resurrection is also for now, in our earthly sojourn. The love God showed in raising Jesus from death transcends time. We take refuge in God's love *now,* not only in the future. God's steadfast love is not bound by time and place.

- In what ways have you seen God's faithfulness in your caregiving story?
- Nothing that belongs to God will go to waste. What might God be redeeming in your life right now?

God who gives steadfast love, may your peace flow like a river around us and carry us ever forward to your heart of compassion. Amen.

TRUST THE LIGHT

*People who have come to know the joy of God do not deny the darkness, but they
choose not to live in it. They claim that the light that shines in the darkness can
be trusted more than the darkness itself and that a little bit of light can dispel a
lot of darkness. They point each other to flashes of light here and there,
and remind each other that they reveal the hidden but real presence of God.
They discover that there are people who heal each other's wounds, forgive each
other's offenses, share their possessions, foster the spirit of community,
celebrate the gifts they have received, and live in constant anticipation
of the full manifestation of God's glory.*

Henri J. M. Nouwen

For it is the God who said, "Let light shine out of darkness,"
who has shone in our hearts to give the light of the knowledge
of the glory of God in the face of Jesus Christ.
—2 CORINTHIANS 4:6

REFLECTION

Many caregivers find themselves in that role because of a turn of circumstances
beyond their control. A season of shock is followed by a learning curve and
clamoring to keep the balls in the air. While we might not name a season of
caregiving as "light," God's light does shine. In a dark space, even a single candle
brings comfort and hope—and the possibility of discovering someone else who
shares the space with whom we can lock arms on the path forward.

- What circumstances or individuals have pointed you toward flashes of
  light in dark times?

- As you live in expectation of God's glory, in what ways is it already shining
  in your circumstances?

*God who shines in our hearts, lighten the way. Remove the fear and dread of
darkness. Point us toward one another as bearers of your light. Amen.*

LIFE THAT TRANSCENDS DEATH

We all have dreams about the perfect life: a life without pain, sadness, conflict or war. The spiritual challenge is to experience glimpses of this perfect life right in the middle of our many struggles. By embracing the reality of our mortal life, we can get in touch with the eternal life that has been sown there. Only by facing our mortality can we come in contact with the life that transcends death. Our imperfections open for us the vision of the perfect life that God in and through Jesus has promised us.

Henri J. M. Nouwen

We are afflicted in every way, but not crushed; perplexed, but not driven to despair; persecuted, but not forsaken; struck down, but not destroyed; always carrying in the body the death of Jesus, so that the life of Jesus may also be made visible in our bodies. For while we live, we are always being given up to death for Jesus' sake, so that the life of Jesus may be made visible in our mortal flesh. So death is at work in us, but life in you.

—2 CORINTHIANS 4:8–12

REFLECTION

The mortal and eternal commingle, constantly reminding us that we live in the in-between. Some days the mortal drags us down, while on others the eternal lifts us up. We must be careful not to put the two experiences in separate realms. If we do, we may fail to see how even our struggles are the soil in which the life of Jesus will grow in us. God is reaping the eternal in our lives now even as paradox surrounds us.

- If you were to write a description of your life similar to today's Scripture passage, what would you include?
- How has being a caregiver shaped your vision of the perfect life?

God who gives eternal life, teach us to recognize it amid the confusion of being afflicted, but not beaten down. May we carry the life of Jesus so your love is made known. Amen.

ADORING YOUR LORD

Once, I had the opportunity of meeting Mother Theresa of Calcutta. I was
struggling with many things and decided to use the occasion to ask Mother
Theresa's advice. As soon as we sat down I started explaining all my problems
and difficulties—trying to convince her of how complicated it all was! When after
ten minutes I finally became silent, Mother Theresa looked at me quietly and said,
"When you spend one hour a day adoring your Lord and never do anything
which you know is wrong, you will be fine!" She punctured my big balloon
of complex self-complaints and pointed me far beyond myself to the place of real
healing. In fact, I was so stunned by her answer that I didn't feel any desire
or need to continue the conversation. I knew that she had spoken the truth
and that I had the rest of my life to live it.

Henri J. M. Nouwen

Ascribe to the Lord the glory due his name;
   bring an offering, and come before him.
Worship the Lord in holy splendor.
   —1 CHRONICLES 16:29

REFLECTION

Caregiving can be a complex experience and often includes a precarious balance
of tasks, resources, time, and emotions. But even amid the calling to embrace
the gift of caring, we may perceive—or create—a story of greater complexity
than necessary. When we start to feel overwhelmed, it may be that it is time to
step back and consider again the essential truths of our calling and find ourselves
once again at the feet of Jesus adoring our Lord.

- What signs in your life might point you to the needed restoration that
  comes through worship?

- In what ways might your caregiving be an offering to the Lord?

God who calls us to adoration, help us to put aside our desire to complicate the
beauty of your calling and simply to offer ourselves to you with whole hearts. Amen.

A NEW EARTH

*As long as we live on this earth, our lives as Christians must be marked by
compassion. The vision of a new heaven and a new earth makes us share one
another's burdens, carry our crosses together, and unite for a better world. In the
new city God will live among us, but each time two or three gather in the name of
Jesus he is already in our midst. In the new city all tears will be wiped away,
but each time people eat bread and drink wine in his memory, smiles appear on
strained faces. In the new city the whole creation will be made new, but each time
prison walls are broken down, poverty is dispelled, and wounds are carefully
attended, the old earth is already giving way to the new. This is the foundation
of our faith, the basis of our hope, and the source of our love.*

Henri J. M. Nouwen

"See, the home of God is among mortals.
He will dwell with them;
they will be his peoples,
and God himself will be with them;
he will wipe every tear from their eyes.
Death will be no more;
mourning and crying and pain will be no more."

—REVELATION 21:3–4

REFLECTION

We do not merely wait for God's redeeming work to make a new heaven and a
new earth; we also participate in it by offering ourselves to one another in healing
compassion. The call to caregiving, rooted as it is in knowing that both we and
the ones we care for are God's beloved, is both a picture of the new heaven and
earth and an experience of it that keeps our hearts expecting God's work in us.

- What parts of your caregiving experience make you yearn for the new
  heaven and earth?
- What parts of caregiving give you glimpses of the fullness of God's redeeming
  work?

*God who makes all things new, wipe our tears. Bend our hearts
toward your redeeming love, which triumphs over all. Amen.*

NOTES
Cited words authored by Henri J. M. Nouwen.

WEEK 1

Letter   From unpublished correspondence. Henri J. M. Nouwen Literary Archives and Research Collection, St. Michael's College, University of Toronto.

Sunday   *Our Greatest Gift: A Meditation on Dying and Caring* (HarperSanFrancisco, 1994; first paperback. ed.), 51–52.

Monday   "Spiritual Direction," *Reflection* Magazine, Yale Divinity School 78, no. 2 (January, 1981): 6-7.

Tuesday   From unpublished television interview transcript, Cross Current, 1995.

Wednesday   *In the Name of Jesus: Reflections on Christian Leadership* (Crossroad Publishing Company, 1989, citation from 1993 paperback edition), 42-44.

Thursday   *A Spirituality of Caregiving* (Henri Nouwen Legacy Trust, 2011), 26–27.

Friday   *Out of Solitude: Three Meditations on the Christian Life* (Ave Maria Press, 1974, citation from 2004 edition), 37–38.

Saturday   *Out of Solitude: Three Meditations on the Christian Life* (Ave Maria Press, 1974, citation from 2004 ed.), 39–40.

WEEK 2

Letter   From unpublished correspondence dated November 2, 1989. Henri J. M. Nouwen Literary Archives and Research Collection, St. Michael's College, University of Toronto.

Sunday   *Compassion: A Reflection on the Christian Life* (Doubleday/Image, 1983), 4, 14.

Monday   *The Way of the Heart: Desert Spirituality and Contemporary Ministry* (HarperCollins, 1981), 33.

Tuesday   *Our Greatest Gift: A Meditation on Dying and Caring* (HarperSanFrancisco, 1994; citation from first paperback ed., 1995), 55–56.

Wednesday   *Our Greatest Gift: A Meditation on Dying and Caring* (HarperSanFrancisco, 1994; citation from first paperback. ed., 1995), 56–57.

Thursday   *Compassion: A Reflection on the Christian Life* (Doubleday/Image, 1983), 15.

Friday   *Lifesigns: Intimacy, Fecundity, and Ecstasy in Christian Perspective* (Image/Doubleday, 1986), 60.

Saturday   *Can You Drink the Cup?* (Ave Maria Press, 1996), 81-82.

WEEK 3

Letter	From unpublished correspondence dated August 11, 1981. Henri J. M. Nouwen Archives and Research Collection, St. Michael's College, University of Toronto.
Sunday	Excerpt from an unpublished manuscript, included in *The Only Necessary Thing: Living a Prayerful Life* (Crossroad Publishing Company, 1999), 204–205.
Monday	*The Return of the Prodigal Son: A Story of Homecoming* (Doubleday, 1992; citation from Doubleday/Image, paperback ed. 1994), 113, 117–118.
Tuesday	*Compassion: A Reflection on the Christian Life* (Doubleday/ Image, 1983), 32.
Wednesday	*Bread for the Journey: A Daybook of Wisdom and Faith* (HarperSanFrancisco, 1997), February 1.
Thursday	*Life of the Beloved: Spiritual Living in a Secular World* (Crossroad Publishing Company, 1992; 10th Anniversary ed., 2002), 89–90.
Friday	*Bread for the Journey: A Daybook of Wisdom and Faith* (HarperSanFrancisco, 1997), March 13.
Saturday	*The Selfless Way of Christ: Downward Mobility and the Spiritual Life* (Orbis Books, 2007; citation from second edition, 2009), 58–60.

WEEK 4

Letter	From unpublished correspondence dated November 8, 1986. Henri J. M. Nouwen Literary Archives and Research Collection, St. Michael's College, University of Toronto.
Sunday	*A Cry for Mercy: Prayers from the Genesee* (Doubleday/Image, 1981; citation from Image paperback ed., 1983) 109.
Monday	*The Selfless Way of Christ: Downward Mobility and the Spiritual Life* (Orbis Books, 2007; citation from second ed., 2009), 86–87.
Tuesday	*The Selfless Way of Christ: Downward Mobility and the Spiritual Life* (Orbis Books, 2007; citation from second ed., 2009) 87–89.
Wednesday	*A Cry for Mercy: Prayers from the Genesee* (Doubleday/Image, 1981; citation from Image paperback ed., 1983), 141.
Thursday	*A Cry for Mercy: Prayers from the Genesee* (Doubleday/Image, 1981; citation from Image paperback ed., 1983), 149.
Friday	"Prayer Embraces the World," *Maryknoll Magazine*, April 1985, 17–21.
Saturday	*Bread for the Journey: A Daybook of Wisdom and Faith* (HarperSanFrancisco, 1997), February 5.

WEEK 5

Letter	From unpublished correspondence. Henri J. M. Nouwen Literary Archives and Research Collection, St. Michael's College, University of Toronto.

Sunday	*The Genesee Diary: Report from a Trappist Monastery* (Doubleday, 1976; Image paperback ed., March 1981), 128–129, September 2.
Monday	From an unpublished address to caregivers at St. Joseph's Hospital. Hamilton, Ontario, 1994.
Tuesday	*Here and Now: Living in the Spirit* (Crossroad Publishing Company, 1994; 1999 ed.), 136–137.
Wednesday	*Bread for the Journey: A Daybook of Wisdom and Faith* (HarperSanFrancisco, 1997), January 8.
Thursday	*Aging: The Fulfillment of Life* (Doubleday/Image, 1974; citation from Image paperback ed., November 1990), 95.
Friday	From the unpublished address "Hope for History." Henri Nouwen Literary Archives, Kelly Library, St. Michael's College, University of Toronto.
Saturday	*Bread for the Journey: A Daybook of Wisdom and Faith* (HarperSanFrancisco, 1997), January 11.

WEEK 6

Letter	From unpublished correspondence dated February 24, 1993. Henri J. M. Nouwen Literary Archives and Research Collection, St. Michael's College, University of Toronto.
Sunday	*Our Greatest Gift: A Meditation on Dying and Caring* (HarperSanFrancisco, 1994; citation from first paperback ed., 1995), 103–104.
Monday	*Bread for the Journey: A Daybook of Wisdom and Faith* (HarperSanFrancisco, 1997), February 10.
Tuesday	*Our Greatest Gift: A Meditation on Dying and Caring* (HarperSanFrancisco, 1994; citation from first paperback edition, 1995), 108–109.
Wednesday	*The Return of the Prodigal Son: A Story of Homecoming* (Doubleday, 1992; citation from Doubleday/Image, paperback ed., 1994), 117.
Thursday	*Bread for the Journey: A Daybook of Wisdom and Faith* (HarperSanFrancisco, 1997), February 26.
Friday	*Here and Now: Living in the Spirit* (Crossroad Publishing Company, 1994; citation from 1999 ed.), 88.
Saturday	*Compassion: A Reflection on the Christian Life* (Doubleday/Image, 1983), 134–135.

PERMISSIONS

Grateful acknowledgement is made for permission to reprint the following excerpts from previously published and unpublished works by Henri J. M. Nouwen.

Unpublished material written by Henri J. M. Nouwen courtesy of the Henri Nouwen Legacy Trust and the Henri J. M. Nouwen Archives and Research Collection, University of St Michael's College, Toronto, Ontario, Canada.

Seven excerpts (973 words) from *Bread for the Journey: A Daybook of Wisdom and Faith* by Henri J. M. Nouwen, copyright © 1997 by the Henri Nouwen Legacy Trust. Reprinted by permission of HarperCollins Publishers.

Five excerpts (704 words) from *Our Greatest Gift: A Meditation on Dying and Caring* by Henri J. M. Nouwen, copyright © 1994 by Henri J. M. Nouwen. Reprinted by permission of HarperCollins Publishers.

One Excerpt (79 words) from *The Way of the Heart* by Henri J. M. Nouwen, copyright © 1981 by Henri J. M. Nouwen. Reprinted by permission of HarperCollins Publishers.

Excerpts from *Here and Now* by Henri Nouwen, copyright © 1994 Henri J. M. Nouwen. Used with permission of Crossroad Publishing Company.

Excerpts from *In the Name of Jesus: Reflections on Christian Leadership*, copyright © 1989 Henri J. M. Nouwen. Used by permission of the Crossroad Publishing Company.

Excerpts from *Life of the Beloved: Spiritual Living in a Secular World*, copyright © 1992 by Henri J. M. Nouwen. Used by permission of the Crossroad Publishing Company.

Excerpts from *The Only Necessary Thing: Living a Prayerful Life*, copyright © 1999 by the Henri J. M. Nouwen Legacy Trust with Wendy Greer. Used by permission of the Crossroad Publishing Company.

Excerpts from *Can You Drink the Cup?* By Henri J. M. Nouwen. Copyright © 1996, 2006 by Ave Maria Press, Inc., P.O. Box 428, Notre Dame, IN 46556, www.avemariapress.com. Used with permission of the publisher.

Excerpts from *Out of Solitude: Three Meditations on the Christian Life*, by Henri J. M. Nouwen. Copyright © 1974, 2004 by Ave Maria Press, Inc., P.O. Box 428, Notre Dame, IN 46556, www.avemariapress.com. Used with permission of the publisher.

Excerpts from *A Cry for Mercy: Prayers from the Genesee by Henri J. M. Nouwen*, copyright © 1981 by Henri J. M. Nouwen. Used by permission of Doubleday, an imprint of Knopf Doubleday Publishing Group, a division of Penguin Random House LLC. All rights reserved.

Excerpts from *Aging: The Fulfillment of Life* by Henri J. M. Nouwen and Walter J. Gaffney, copyright renewed ©2002 by Sue Mosteller, Executor of the Estate of Henri J. M. Nouwen. Used by permission of Doubleday, an imprint of Knopf Doubleday Publishing Group, a division of Penguin Random House LLC. All rights reserved.

BOOKS BY
HENRI J. M. NOUWEN

Adam: God's Beloved
Aging
Behold the Beauty of the Lord
Beyond the Mirror
Bread for the Journey
Can you Drink the Cup?
Clowning in Rome
Compassion
Creative Ministry
A Cry for Mercy
Encounters with Merton
Finding My Way Home
Finding Our Sacred Centre
The Genesee Diary
Gracias: A Latin American Journal
Heart Speaks to Heart
Here and Now
Home Tonight
In Memoriam
In the Name of Jesus
The Inner Voice of Love
Intimacy
Jesus and Mary
A Letter of Consolation
Letters to Marc About Jesus
Life of the Beloved
Lifesigns
The Living Reminder

Love, Henri: Letters on
  the Spiritual Life
Love in a Fearful Land
Making All Things New
The Only Necessary Thing
Our Great Gift
Out of Solitude
Path of Freedom
Path of Peace
Path of Power
Path of Waiting
Peacework
Reaching Out
The Return of the Prodigal Son
The Road to Daybreak
Sabbatical Journey
Seeds of Hope
The Selfless Way of Christ
Show Me the Way
A Sorrow Shared
A Spirituality of Caregiving
A Spirituality of Fundraising
A Spirituality of Living
Thomas Merton: Contemplative Critic
Walk with Jesus
The Way of the Heart
With Open Hands
With Burning Hearts
The Wounded Healer

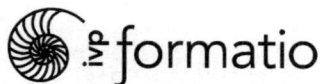

IVP formatio

The nautilus is one of the sea's oldest creatures. Beginning with a tight center, its remarkable growth pattern can be seen in the ever-enlarging chambers that spiral outward. The nautilus in the IVP Formatio logo symbolizes deep inward work of spiritual formation that begins rooted in our souls and then opens to the world as we experience spiritual transformation. The shell takes on a stunning pearlized appearance as it ages and forms in much the same way as the souls of those who devote themselves to spiritual practice. Formatio books draw on the ancient wisdom of the saints and the early church as well as the rich resources of Scripture, applying tradition to the needs of contemporary life and practice.

Within each of us is a longing to be in God's presence. Formatio books call us into our deepest desires and help us to become our true selves in the light of God's grace.

VISIT
ivpress.com/formatio
*to see all of the books in the
line and to sign up for the
IVP Formatio newsletter.*